The Ultimate Comfort Food Guide for A Delicious Lunch

Super tasty and easy lunch comfort food recipes

Robert Wagon

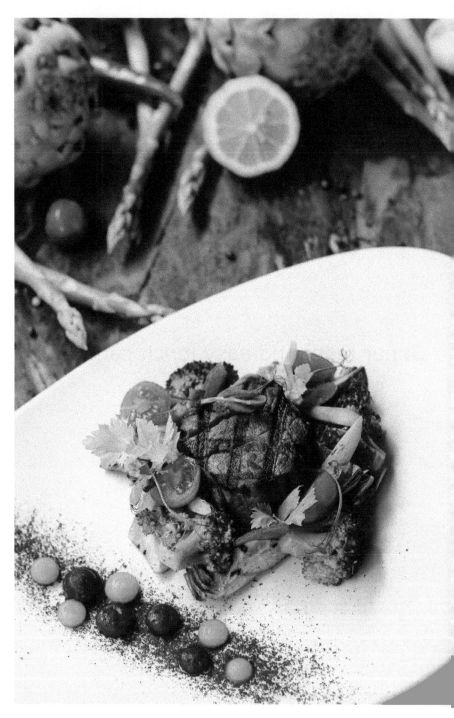

professional advice. The content within this book has been derived from various sources. Please consult a licensed professional before attempting any techniques outlined in this book.

By reading this document, the reader agrees that under no circumstances is the author responsible for any losses, direct or indirect, which are incurred as a result of the use of information contained within this document, including, but not limited to, — errors, omissions, or inaccuracies.

Table of contents

Mushroom Pork Brisket

Preparation Time: 5 minutes | Cooking Time: 40 minutes

Serving: 10

Ingredients:

3 cloves garlic, minced

2 cups red wine

4 pounds pork brisket

3 tablespoons peppercorn

1 tablespoon butter

1 cup mushrooms, cut into slices

2 cups chicken broth

Pepper and salt as needed

Directions:

Take your Pressure Pot and place it over a dry kitchen platform.

Open the lid and add the above-mentioned ingredients. Stir the ingredients gently to mix them.

Lock the top lid and make sure that the valve is sealed properly.

Select "Meat/Stew" cooking function. Set the cooking time to 40 minutes.

Your Pressure Pot will start building the pressure and begin the cooking cycle after a sufficient level of pressure is reached.

After the cooking time is over, press the "Cancel" setting, and then press "NPR" for the natural release of the internal pressure. It takes around 10 minutes to release the pressure naturally.

Open the top lid and slice the meat. Transfer the meat and the sauce to your serving bowls.

Serve and enjoy the recipe.

Nutrition:

Calories 487, Total Carbohydrates 13g, Fiber 1g, Saturated Fat 19g, Trans Fat 0g, Protein 32g, Sodium 638g.

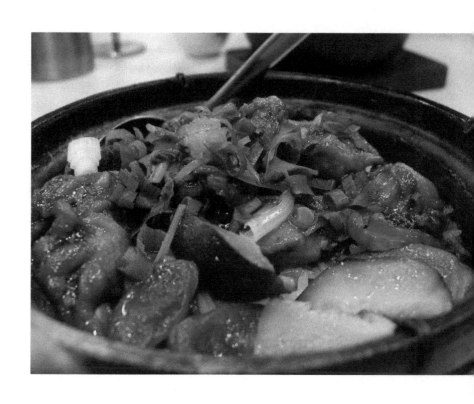

Creamy Pork Noodles

Preparation Time: 5 minutes | Cooking Time: 40 minutes

Serving: 4

Ingredients:

2 stalks of celery, diced

1 onion, diced

1-pound pork loin, cut in strips

3 carrots, chopped

½ cup sour cream

2 cups chicken broth

1 tablespoon Dijon mustard

1 package egg noodles, cooked

Directions:

Take your Pressure Pot and place it over a dry kitchen platform.

Open the lid and add the above-mentioned ingredients except for the noodles. Stir the ingredients gently to mix with each other.

Lock the top lid and make sure that the valve is sealed properly.

Select "Meat/Stew" cooking function. Set the cooking time to 40 minutes.

Your Pressure Pot will start building the pressure and begin the cooking cycle after a sufficient level of pressure is reached.

After the cooking time is over, press the "Cancel" setting, and then press "NPR" for the natural release of the internal pressure. It takes around 10 minutes to release the pressure naturally.

Open the top lid and transfer the meat to your bowls.

Serve with the cooked noodles on top and enjoy the recipe.

Nutrition:

Calories 596, Total Carbohydrates 16g, Fiber 2g, Saturated Fat 11g, Trans Fat 0g, Protein 76g, Sodium 423g.

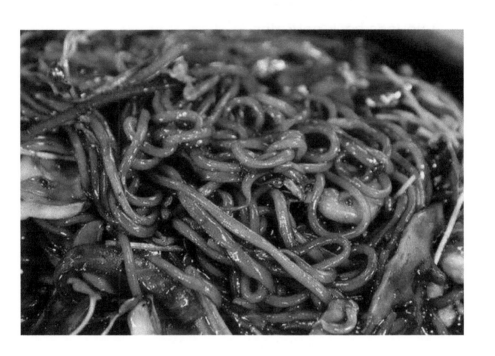

Sweet BBQ Pork

Preparation Time: 10 minutes | Cooking Time: 95 minutes

Serving: 4

Ingredients:

½ teaspoon ground cumin

2 pounds back pork ribs

2 tablespoons apple cider vinegar

½ teaspoon black pepper

2 cups apple juice

1 tablespoon liquid smoke

1 teaspoon salt

½ teaspoon brown sugar

1 tablespoon Worcestershire sauce

½ teaspoon garlic powder

¼ cup BBQ sauce

¼ cup tomato ketchup

Directions:

Combine the salt, pepper, brown sugar, cumin, and garlic powder in a mixing bowl.

Add the pork to the mixture and mix well. Set aside to marinate for 40 minutes.

Take your Pressure Pot and place it over a dry kitchen platform.

Open the lid and add the apple cider vinegar, liquid smoke, marinated pork, marinade leftovers, and apple juice. Stir the ingredients gently to combine with each other.

Lock the top lid and make sure that the valve is sealed properly.

Select "Meat/Stew" cooking function. Set the cooking time to 25 minutes.

Your Pressure Pot will start building the pressure and begin the cooking cycle after a sufficient level of pressure is reached.

After the cooking time is over, press the "Cancel" setting, and then press "NPR" for the natural release of the internal pressure. It takes around 10 minutes to release the pressure naturally.

Open the top lid and mix in the BBQ sauce, ketchup, and Worcestershire sauce.

Close the lid and let the flavors mix up and infuse for Set aside 15 minutes.

Transfer the meat to your serving plates and pour the remaining sauce on top.

Serve with a side of your choice and enjoy the recipe.

Nutrition:

Calories 674, Total Carbohydrates 24g, Fiber 6g, Saturated Fat 27g, Trans Fat 0g, Protein 36g, Sodium 1124g.

Asian-Style Garlic Pork

Preparation Time: 5 minutes | Cooking Time: 45 minutes

Serving: 8-9

Ingredients:

3 stalks of green onions, chopped

4 cloves of garlic, minced

4 stars anise

4 cloves

3 pounds of pork belly

1 thumb-size ginger, grated

½ cup brown sugar

½ cup of soy sauce

½ cup soy paste

½ cup Shaoxing wine

Directions:

Take your Pressure Pot and place it over a dry kitchen platform.

Open the lid and add the above-mentioned ingredient**s** .

Stir the ingredients gently to combine with each other.

Lock the top lid and make sure that the valve is sealed properly.

Select "Meat/Stew" cooking function. Set the cooking time to 45 minutes.

Your Pressure Pot will start building the pressure and begin the cooking cycle after a sufficient level of pressure is reached.

After the cooking time is over, press the "Cancel" setting, and then press "NPR" for the natural release of the internal pressure. It takes around 10 minutes to release the pressure naturally.

Open the top lid and slice the meat and transfer to your serving bowls.

Serve with some rice noodles and enjoy the recipe.

Nutrition:

Calories 723, Total Carbohydrates 16g, Fiber 0.5g, Saturated Fat 32g, Trans Fat 0g, Protein 16g, Sodium 368g.

Chinese Moo Shu Cabbage pork

Preparation Time: 5 minutes | Cooking Time: 30 minutes

Serving: 4

Ingredients:

1 tablespoon minced garlic

1-pound pork chops, cut into strips

¼ cup beef broth

2 teaspoons sesame oil

1 onion, chopped

3 tablespoons soy sauce

1/3 cup hoisin sauce

1 bag of shredded cabbages

2 tablespoons cornstarch + 2 tablespoons water

Directions:

Take your Pressure Pot and place it over a dry kitchen platform.

Open the lid and select the "Sauté" cooking function.

Add the oil, garlic, and onions into the pot; cook to soften for 2-3 minutes

Add in the pork strips and sauté for 4-5 minutes.

Pour in the broth, soy sauce, and hoisin sauce; gently stir.

Lock the top lid and make sure that the valve is sealed properly.

Select "Meat/Stew" cooking function. Set the cooking time to 25 minutes.

Your Pressure Pot will start building the pressure and begin the cooking cycle after a sufficient level of pressure is reached.

After the cooking time is over, press the "Cancel" setting, and then press "NPR" for the natural release of the internal pressure. It takes around 10 minutes to release the pressure naturally.

Open the top lid.

Mix in the shredded cabbages and cornstarch slurry.

Simmer using the "Sauté" cooking function until the sauce thickens.

Serve warm.

Nutrition:

Calories 361, Total Carbohydrates 18g, Fiber 2g, Saturated Fat 9g, Trans Fat 0g, Protein 31g, Sodium 486g.

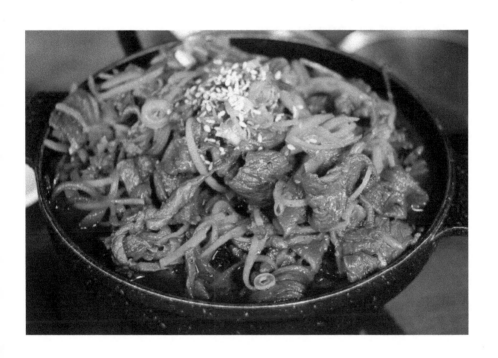

Cranberry Rosemary Pork Chops

Preparation Time: 5 minutes | Cooking Time: 60 minutes

Serving: 5-6

Ingredients:

1 onion, diced

½ cup of orange juice

¼ cup maple syrup

4 tablespoons coconut oil

1 ½ pound pork chops, bone-in

1 ½ teaspoon cinnamon

1 teaspoon garlic cloves

1/3 cup cranberries

2 teaspoons rosemary, fresh

Pepper and salt as per your taste preference

Directions:

Take your Pressure Pot and place it over a dry kitchen platform.

Open the lid and select the "Sauté" cooking function.

Add the oil and meat to the pot; cook for 2 minutes to brown.

Add the remaining ingredients; gently stir.

Lock the top lid and make sure that the valve is sealed properly.

Select "Meat/Stew" cooking function. Set the cooking time to 60 minutes.

Your Pressure Pot will start building the pressure and begin the cooking cycle after a sufficient level of pressure is reached.

After the cooking time is over, press the "Cancel" setting, and then press "NPR" for the natural release of the internal pressure. It takes around 10 minutes to release the pressure naturally.

Open the top lid and transfer the meat to your serving plates and pour the sauce on top.

Serve and enjoy the recipe.

Nutrition:

Calories 323, Total Carbohydrates 10g, Fiber 0.5g, Saturated Fat 12g, Trans Fat 0g, Protein 45g, Sodium 364g.

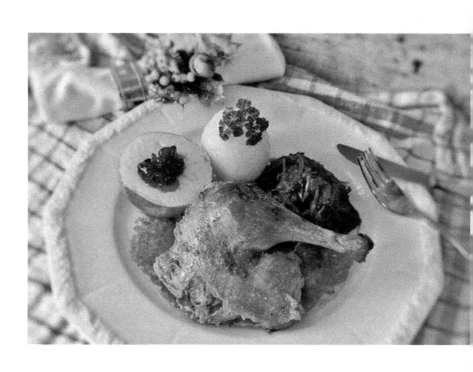

Coconut Lentils

Preparation Time: 5 minutes | Cooking Time: 30 minutes

Serving: 4

Ingredients:

1 1/2 cups lentils

15 oz can coconut milk

2 tbsp tomato paste

15 oz tomato sauce

1 tsp dried oregano

1 tsp dried basil

1/4 cup water

1/4 tsp garlic salt

Directions:

Add all ingredients into the Pressure Pot and stir well.

Seal pot with lid and cook on high for 20 minutes.

Release pressure using the quick-release method than open the lid.

Stir well and serve over rice.

Nutrition:

Calories 332, Carbohydrates 35.9g, Protein 15g, Fat 15g, Sugar 4.7g, Sodium, 389mg.

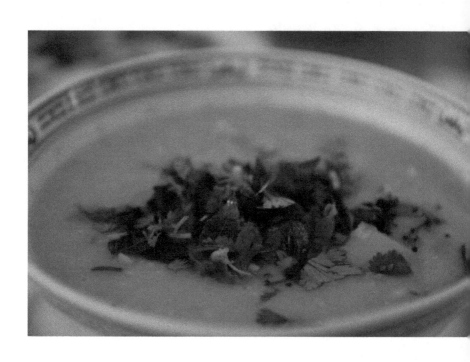

Rosemary Potatoes

Preparation Time: 5 minutes | Cooking Time: 30 minutes

Serving: 4

Ingredients:

1 lb potatoes, scrubbed and sliced

1/4 tsp rosemary, dried

2 garlic cloves, sliced

1 tbsp olive oil

Salt

Directions:

Pour 1 cup of water into the Pressure Pot and place the steamer basket into the pot.

Add sliced potatoes to the steamer basket.

Seal pot with lid and cook on high for 4 minutes.

Release pressure using the quick-release method than open the lid.

Add olive oil, garlic, and rosemary into the oven-safe dish and microwave for 1 minute.

Add sliced potatoes into the dish and stir to coat.

Serve and enjoy.

Nutrition:

Calories 111, Carbohydrates 18g, Protein 2g, Fat 0.5g, Sugar 1.3g, Sodium 46mg.

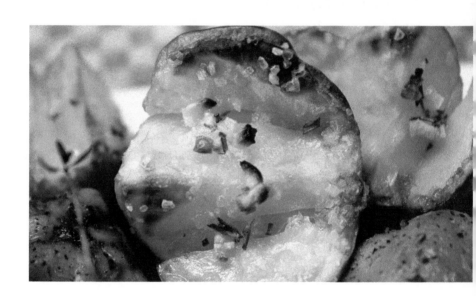

Crispy Okra

Preparation Time: 10 minutes | Cooking Time: 10 minutes | Servings: 2

Ingredients:

3 cups okra, wash and dry

1 tsp cumin powder

1 tsp fresh lemon juice

1 tsp red chili powder

3 tbsp gram flour

1/2 tsp coriander powder

Salt

Directions:

Cut top of okra then makes a deep horizontal cut in each okra and set aside.

In a bowl, combine gram flour, lemon juice, chili powder, coriander powder, cumin powder, mango powder, and salt.

Add little water in gram flour mixture and make a thick batter.

Spray Pressure Pot multi-level air fryer basket with cooking spray.

Fill the batter in each okra and place it into the air fryer basket and place the basket into the Pressure Pot.

Seal pot with air fryer lid and select air fry mode then set the temperature to 390° F and timer for 10 minutes. Serve and enjoy.

Nutrition:

Calories 102, Fat 1.3g, Carbohydrates 17.4g, Sugar 3.3g, Protein 5.2g, Cholesterol 0mg.

Garlic Mushrooms

Preparation Time: 10 minutes | Cooking Time: 25 minutes | Servings: 2

Ingredients:

1 lbs mushrooms, wash, dry, and cut into quarter

1/4 tsp garlic powder

1 tsp herb de Provence

1/2 tbsp olive oil

1 tbsp white vermouth

Directions:

Add all ingredients to the bowl and toss well.

Spray Pressure Pot multi-level air fryer basket with cooking spray.

Add mushrooms into the air fryer basket and place basket into the Pressure Pot.

Seal pot with air fryer lid and select air fry mode then set the temperature to 350° F and timer for 25 minutes. Stir halfway through.

Serve and enjoy.

Nutrition:

Calories 92, Fat 4.4g, Carbohydrates 7.9g, Sugar 4g, Protein 7.7g, Cholesterol 0mg.

Crispy Zucchini Fries

Preparation Time: 10 minutes | Cooking Time: 15 minutes | Servings: 2

Ingredients:

2 medium zucchinis, cut into French fries' shape

1 tbsp water

1/2 tbsp olive oil

2 tbsp cornstarch

Salt

Directions:

Spray Pressure Pot multi-level air fryer basket with cooking spray.

Add all ingredients into the bowl and mix well.

Place coated zucchini fries into the air fryer basket and place the basket into the Pressure Pot.

Seal pot with air fryer lid and select air fry mode then set the temperature to 390° F and timer for 15 minutes. Stir halfway through.

Serve and enjoy.

Nutrition:

Calories 92, Fat 3.9g, Carbohydrates 13.9g, Sugar 3.4g, Protein 2.4g, Cholesterol 0mg.

Tasty & Crispy Tofu

Preparation Time: 10 minutes | Cooking Time: 20 minutes | Servings: 4

Ingredients:

1 block firm tofu, pressed and cut into 1-inch cubes

1 tsp vinegar

2 tbsp soy sauce

1 tbsp corn flour

2 tsp sesame oil

Directions:

In a bowl, toss tofu with oil, vinegar, and soy sauce and let sit for 15 minutes.

Toss marinated tofu with corn flour.

Spray Pressure Pot multi-level air fryer basket with cooking spray.

Add tofu into the air fryer basket and place basket into the Pressure Pot.

Seal pot with air fryer lid and select air fry mode then set the temperature to 370° F and timer for 20 minutes. Stir halfway through.

Serve and enjoy.

Nutrition:

Calories 47, Fat 3.3g, Carbohydrates 2.4g, Sugar 0.3g, Protein 2.5g, Cholesterol 0mg.

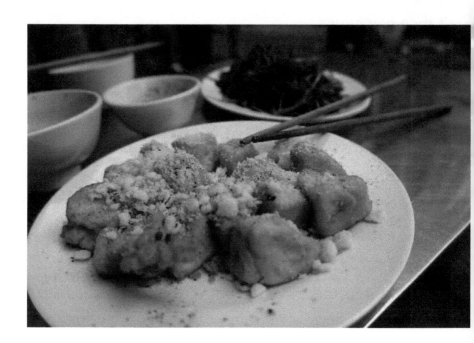

Simple Green Beans

Preparation Time: 5 minutes | Cooking Time: 10 minutes | Servings: 2

Ingredients:

8 oz green beans, trimmed and cut in half

1 tbsp tamari

1 tsp sesame oil

Directions:

Add all ingredients into the large mixing bowl and toss well.

Spray Pressure Pot multi-level air fryer basket with cooking spray.

Transfer green beans into the air fryer basket and place basket into the Pressure Pot.

Seal pot with air fryer lid and select air fry mode then set the temperature to 400° F and timer for 10 minutes. Stir halfway through.

Serve and enjoy.

Nutrition:

Calories 61, Fat 2.4g, Carbohydrates 8.6g, Sugar 1.7g, Protein 3g, Cholesterol 0mg.

Flavors Eggplant

Preparation Time: 10 minutes | Cooking Time: 12 minutes | Servings: 2

Ingredients:

1 eggplant, washed and cubed

1/4 tsp oregano

1 tbsp olive oil

1/2 tsp garlic powder

1/4 tsp marjoram

Directions:

Add all ingredients into the mixing bowl and toss well.

Spray Pressure Pot multi-level air fryer basket with cooking spray.

Transfer eggplant into the air fryer basket and place basket into the Pressure Pot.

Seal pot with air fryer lid and select air fry mode then set the temperature to 390° F and timer for 12 minutes. Stir halfway through.

Serve and enjoy.

Nutrition:

Calories 120, Fat 7.5g, Carbohydrates 14.2g, Sugar 7.1g, Protein 2.4g, Cholesterol 0mg.

Air Fried Bell Peppers

Preparation Time: 5 minutes | Cooking Time: 8 minutes | Servings: 3

Ingredients:

3 cups bell peppers, cut into chunks

1/4 tsp garlic powder

1 tsp olive oil

Pepper

Salt

Directions:

Add all ingredients into the mixing bowl and toss well.

Spray Pressure Pot multi-level air fryer basket with cooking spray.

Transfer bell peppers into the air fryer basket and place basket into the Pressure Pot.

Seal pot with air fryer lid and select air fry mode then set the temperature to 360° F and timer for 8 minutes. Stir halfway through.

Serve and enjoy.

Nutrition:

Calories 52, Fat 1.9g, Carbohydrates 9.2g, Sugar 6.1g, Protein 1.2g, Cholesterol 0mg.

Tasty Cauliflower & Broccoli

Preparation Time: 10 minutes | Cooking Time: 12 minutes | Servings: 6

Ingredients:

3 cups cauliflower florets

1/2 tsp garlic powder

2 tbsp olive oil

1/4 tsp onion powder

3 cups broccoli florets

1/4 tsp paprika

1/8 tsp pepper

1/4 tsp sea salt

Directions:

Add cauliflower and broccoli into the large bowl. Add remaining ingredients and toss well.

Spray Pressure Pot multi-level air fryer basket with cooking spray.

Transfer broccoli and cauliflower mixture into the air fryer basket and place basket into the Pressure Pot.

Seal pot with air fryer lid and select air fry mode then set the temperature to 380° F and timer for 12 minutes. Stir halfway through.

Serve and enjoy.

Nutrition:

Calories 69, Fat 4.9g, Carbohydrates 6g, Sugar 2.1g, Protein 2.3g, Cholesterol 0mg.

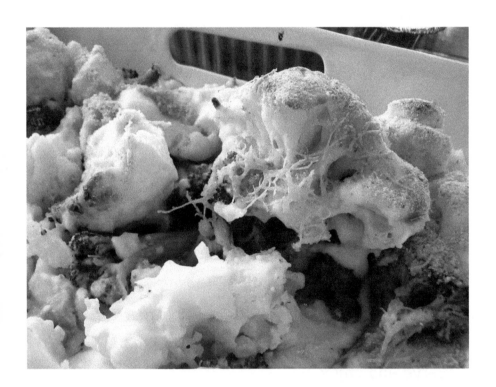

Air Fried Mushrooms

Preparation Time: 5 minutes | Cooking Time: 8 minutes | Servings: 2

Ingredients:

12 button mushrooms, cleaned

1 tsp olive oil

1/4 tsp Pepper

1/4 tsp garlic salt

Directions:

Add all ingredients into the bowl and toss well.

Spray Pressure Pot multi-level air fryer basket with cooking spray.

Transfer mushrooms into the air fryer basket and place basket into the Pressure Pot.

Seal pot with air fryer lid and select air fry mode then set the temperature to 380° F and timer for 8 minutes. Stir halfway through.

Serve and enjoy.

Nutrition:

Calories 45, Fat 2.7g, Carbohydrates 4g, Sugar 1.9g, Protein 3.5g, Cholesterol 0mg.

Flavorful Lemon Chicken

Preparation time: 10 minutes | Cooking Time: 4 hours 5 minutes | Servings: 4

Ingredients:

20 oz chicken breasts, skinless, boneless, and cut into pieces

1 tsp dried parsley

2 tbsp olive oil

2 tbsp butter

3 tbsp flour

1/4 cup chicken broth

1/2 cup fresh lemon juice

1/8 tsp dried thyme fla

1/4 tsp dried basil

1/2 tsp dried oregano

1 tsp salt

Directions:

In a bowl, toss chicken with flour.

Heat butter and oil in a pan over medium-high heat.

Add chicken to the pan and sear until brown.

Transfer chicken into the inner pot of Pressure Pot duo crisp.

Add remaining ingredients on top of chicken.

Seal the pot with a pressure-cooking lid and select slow cook mode and cook on low for 4 hours.

Serve and enjoy.

Nutrition:

Calories 412, Fat 23.7g, Carbohydrates 5.3g, Sugar 0.7g, Protein 42.3g, Cholesterol 141mg.

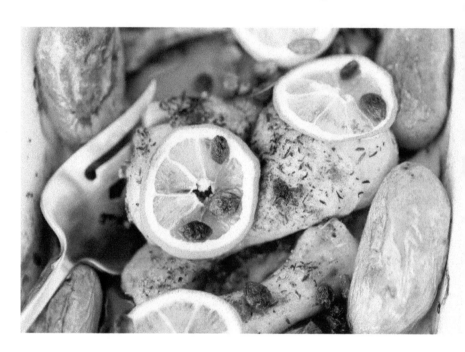

Dijon Chicken

Preparation time: 10 minutes | Cooking Time: 50 minutes | Servings: 4

Ingredients:

1 1/2 lbs. chicken thighs, skinless and boneless

2 tbsp Dijon mustard

1/4 cup French mustard

4 tbsp maple syrup

2 tsp olive oil

Directions:

In a large bowl, mix maple syrup, olive oil, Dijon mustard, and French mustard.

Add chicken to the bowl and mix until chicken is well coated.

Transfer chicken into the Pressure Pot air fryer basket and place basket in the pot.

Seal the pot with an air fryer lid and select bake mode and cook at 375° F for 45-50 minutes.

Serve and enjoy.

Nutrition:

Calories 401, Fat 15.3g, Carbohydrates 13.8g, Sugar 12g, Protein 49.6g, Cholesterol 151mg.

Mango Chicken

Preparation time: 10 minutes | Cooking Time: 15 minutes | Servings: 2

Ingredients:

2 chicken breasts, skinless and boneless

1 ripe mango, peeled and diced

1/2 tbsp turmeric

1/2 cup chicken broth

2 garlic cloves, minced

1/2 tsp ginger, grated

1 fresh lime juice

1/2 tsp pepper

1/2 tsp salt

Directions:

Add chicken into the inner pot of Pressure Pot duo crisp and top with mango.

Add lime juice, broth, turmeric, pepper, and salt.

Seal the pot with a pressure-cooking lid and cook on high for 15 minutes.

Once done, allow to release pressure naturally. Remove lid.

Shred chicken using a fork and stir well.

Serve and enjoy.

Nutrition:

Calories 407, Fat 12.1g, Carbohydrates 30g, Sugar 23.6g, Protein 45.3g, Cholesterol 130mg.

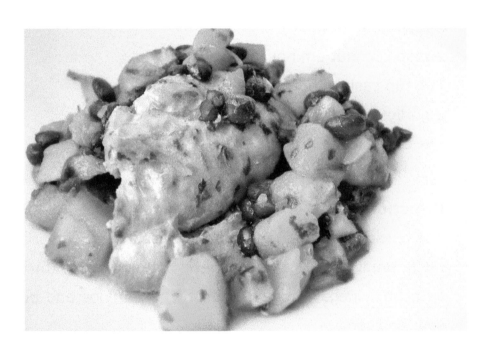

Honey Cashew Butter Chicken

Preparation time: 10 minutes | Cooking Time: 7 minutes | Servings: 3

Ingredients:

1 lb chicken breast, cut into chunks

2 tbsp rice vinegar

2 tbsp honey

2 tbsp coconut aminos

1/4 cup cashew butter

2 garlic cloves, minced

1/4 cup chicken broth

1/2 tbsp sriracha

Directions:

Add chicken into the inner pot of Pressure Pot duo crisp. In a small bowl, mix cashew butter, garlic, broth, sriracha, vinegar, honey, and coconut aminos and pour over chicken.

Seal the pot with a pressure-cooking lid and cook on high for 7 minutes.

Once done, release pressure using a quick release. Remove lid.

Stir well and serve.

Nutrition:

Calories 366, Fat 2.1g, Carbohydrates 20.7g, Sugar 11.6g, Protein 36.4g, Cholesterol 97mg.

Sweet & Tangy Tamarind Chicken

Preparation time: 10 minutes | Cooking Time: 15 minutes | Servings: 4

Ingredients:

2 lbs chicken breasts, skinless, boneless, and cut into pieces

1 tbsp ketchup

1 tbsp vinegar

2 tbsp ginger, grated

1 garlic clove, minced

3 tbsp olive oil

1 tbsp arrowroot powder

1/2 cup tamarind paste

2 tbsp brown sugar

1 tsp salt

Directions:

Add oil into the inner pot of Pressure Pot duo crisp and set the pot on sauté mode.

Add ginger and garlic and sauté for 30 seconds.

Add chicken and sauté for 3-4 minutes.

In a small bowl, mix the tamarind paste, brown sugar, ketchup, vinegar, and salt and pour over chicken and stir well.

Seal the pot with a pressure-cooking lid and cook on high for 8 minutes.

Once done, release pressure using a quick release. Remove lid.

In a small bowl, whisk arrowroot powder with 2 tbsp water and pour it into the pot.

Set pot on sauté mode and cook chicken for 1-2 minutes.

Serve and enjoy.

Nutrition:

Calories 598, Fat 27.6g, Carbohydrates 18.9g, Sugar 14g, Protein 66.4g, Cholesterol 202mg.

Korean chicken wings

Preparation time: 5 minutes | Cooking Time: 10 minutes | Servings: 8

Ingredients:

Wings:

1 tsp. Pepper

1 tsp. Salt

2 pounds of chicken wings

Sauce:

2 packets Splenda

1 tbsp. Minced garlic

1 tbsp. Minced ginger

1 tbsp. Sesame oil

1 tsp. Agave nectar

1 tbsp. Mayo

2 tbsp. Gochujang

Finishing:

¼ c. Chopped green onions

2 tsp. Sesame seeds

Directions:

Preparing the ingredients. Ensure instant crisp air fryer is preheated to 400 degrees.

Line a small pan with foil and place a rack onto the pan, then place into an instant crisp air fryer.

Season wings with pepper and salt and place them onto the rack.

Air frying. Lock the air fryer lid. Set temperature to 160°F and set time to 20 minutes and air fry 20 minutes, turning at 10 minutes.

As chicken air fries, mix all the sauce components.

Once a thermometer says that the chicken has reached 160° F, take out wings and place them into a bowl.

Pour half of the sauce mixture over wings, tossing well to coat.

Put coated wings back into an instant crisp air fryer for 5 minutes or till they reach 165° F.

Remove and sprinkle with green onions and sesame seeds. Dip into the extra sauce.

Nutrition:

Calories 356, Fat 26g, Protein 23g, Sugar 2g.

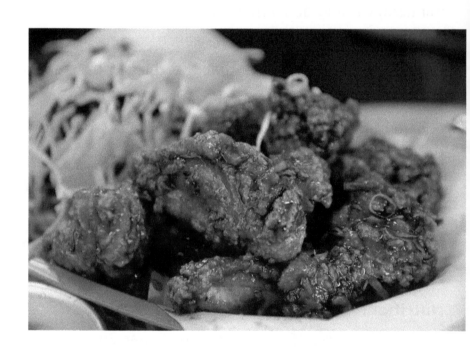

Sweet Carrots

Preparation Time: 10 minutes | Cooking Time: 3 minutes | Servings: 8

Ingredients:

2 lbs carrots, peeled and sliced thickly

3 tbsp raisins

1 tbsp maple syrup

1 tbsp butter

1 cup of water

Pepper

Salt

Directions:

Add water, carrots, and raisins in the inner pot of Pressure Pot duo crisp.

Seal the pot with a pressure-cooking lid and cook on high for 3 minutes.

Once done, release pressure using a quick release. Remove lid.

Drain carrots and transfer to the mixing bowl.

Add butter and maple syrup over carrots and toss well.

Season with pepper and salt.

Serve and enjoy.

Nutrition:

Calories 76, Fat 1.5g, Carbohydrates 15.5g, Sugar 9.1g, Protein 1.1g, Cholesterol 4mg.

Spicy Rice

Preparation Time: 10 minutes | Cooking Time: 3 minutes | Servings: 2

Ingredients:

1 cup rice, long grain

1/4 cup green hot sauce

1/2 cup fresh cilantro, chopped

1/2 avocado flesh

1 1/4 cup vegetable broth

Pepper

Salt

Directions:

Add broth and rice in the inner pot of Pressure Pot duo crisp and stir well.

Seal the pot with a pressure-cooking lid and cook on high for 3 minutes.

Once done, allow to release pressure naturally. Remove lid.

Fluff the rice using a fork.

Add green sauce, avocado, and cilantro in a blender and blend until smooth.

Pour blended mixture into the rice and stir well to combine. Season with pepper and salt.

Serve and enjoy.

Nutrition:

Calories 375, Fat 2.6g, Carbohydrates 75.5g, Sugar 0.6g, Protein 10g, Cholesterol 0mg.

Indian Potato Curry

Preparation Time: 10 minutes | Cooking Time: 7 minutes | Servings: 4

Ingredients:

2 medium potatoes, peeled and chopped

1/2 tsp garam masala

1 Serrano, minced

1/2 cup onion masala

1 tsp cumin seeds

1 1/2 cups water

2 cups fresh peas

2 tbsp olive oil

1/4 tsp pepper

1 tsp salt

Directions:

Add oil into the inner pot of Pressure Pot duo crisp and set pot on sauté mode.

Add Serrano pepper and cumin seeds and sauté for 1-2 minutes.

Add remaining ingredients and stir well.

Seal the pot with a pressure-cooking lid and cook on high for 5 minutes.

Once done, release pressure using a quick release. Remove lid.

Serve and enjoy.

Nutrition:

Calories 244, Fat 9.5g, Carbohydrates 33.4g, Sugar 6.2g, Protein 7.7g.

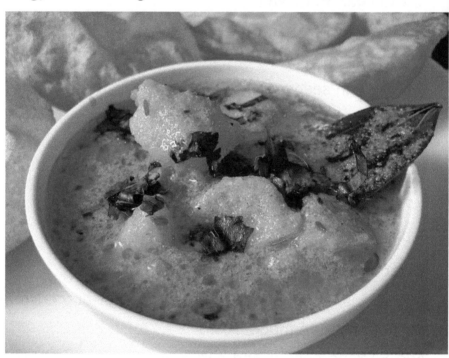

Creamy Squash Apple Mash

Preparation Time: 5 minutes | Cooking Time: 30 minutes

Serving: 4

Ingredients:

1 lb butternut squash, cut into 2" pieces

2 apples, cored and sliced

1 cup of water

2 tbsp coconut oil

1 onion, sliced

1/4 tsp ground cinnamon

1/8 tsp ginger powder

1/4 tsp salt

Directions:

Pour water into the Pressure Pot and place the steamer basket into the pot.

Toss apples, butternut squash, and onion together and put in a steamer basket. Season with salt.

Seal pot with lid and cook on high for 8 minutes.

Release pressure using the quick-release method than open the lid.

Transfer apple and squash mixture into the bowl and mash until smooth.

Add coconut oil, ginger, and cinnamon and mix well to combine.

Serve and enjoy.

Nutrition:

Calories 179, Carbohydrates 31.4g, Protein 1.8g, Fat 7.1g, Sugar 15g, Sodium 156mg.

Parmesan Asparagus

Preparation Time: 5 minutes | Cooking Time: 30 minutes

Serving: 4

Ingredients:

25 asparagus spear ends trimmed and cut into pieces

3 garlic cloves, minced

3 tbsp butter

3 tbsp parmesan cheese, grated

1 cup of water

Directions:

Pour water into the Pressure Pot then place the trivet in the pot.

Place asparagus on foil piece and top with garlic and butter then curve the edges of foil.

Place foil on a trivet. Seal pot with lid and cook on high for 8 minutes.

Release pressure using the quick-release method than open the lid.

Sprinkle with parmesan cheese and serve.

Nutrition:

Calories 232, Carbohydrates 4.6g, Protein 6.7g, Fat 13.2g, Sugar 1.6g, Sodium 309mg.

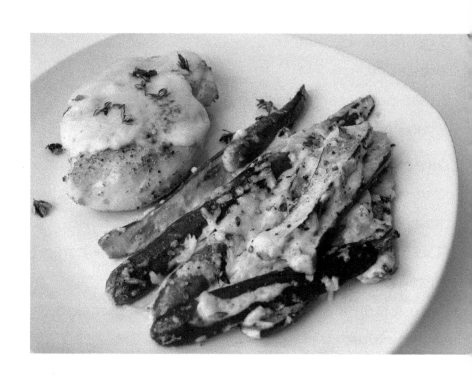

Turnip Mash

Preparation Time: 5 minutes | Cooking Time: 30 minutes

Serving: 4

Ingredients:

4 medium turnips, peeled and diced

1/4 cup sour cream

1/2 cup vegetable broth

1 onion, diced

Pepper

Salt

Directions:

Add turnips, broth, and onion into the Pressure Pot.

Seal pot with lid and cook on high for 5 minutes.

Allow releasing pressure naturally for 10 minutes then release using the quick release method.

Drain turnip well and transfer in mixing bowl and mash turnips until smooth.

Add sour cream and stir well. Season with pepper and salt.

Serve and enjoy.

Nutrition:

Calories 82, Carbohydrates 11g, Protein 2.4g, Fat 3.2g, Sugar 6.3g, Sodium 223mg.

Braised Parsnips

Preparation Time: 5 minutes | Cooking Time: 30 minutes

Serving: 4

Ingredients:

1 1/2 lbs parsnips, peeled and sliced

3 tbsp balsamic vinegar

1/4 cup vegetable broth

2 tbsp maple syrup

1/8 tsp pepper

1/2 tsp salt

Directions:

Add parsnips, vinegar, and broth into the Pressure Pot.

Seal pot with lid and cook on high pressure for 3 minutes.

Release pressure using the quick-release method than open the lid.

Add maple syrup and stir well. Season with pepper and salt.

Serve and enjoy.

Nutrition:

Calories 159, Carbohydrates 37g, Protein 2.4g, Fat 0.6g, Sugar 14.2g, Sodium 357mg.

Turmeric Mushrooms

Preparation Time: 5 minutes | Cooking Time: 30 minutes

Serving: 4

Ingredients:

24 oz Bella mushrooms, sliced

1 tbsp olive oil

3 tbsp water

1/2 tsp mustard seeds

1 tsp cumin seeds

1/4 tsp turmeric powder

3 curry leaves

2 tsp salt

Directions:

Add olive oil into the Pressure Pot and set the pot on sauté mode.

Add cumin seeds and mustard seeds and let them pop.

Add sliced mushrooms, turmeric, curry leaves, and salt. Stir well.

Add water and stir. Seal pot with lid and cook on steam mode for 2 minutes.

Release pressure using the quick-release method than open the lid.

Set Pressure Pot on sauté mode. Stir mushrooms and simmer for 3-4 minutes.

Serve and enjoy.

Nutrition:

Calories 83, Carbohydrates 5.3g, Protein 5.1g, Fat 3.8g, Sugar 0g, Sodium 1164mg.

Pumpkin Spice Butternut Squash

Preparation Time: 5 minutes | Cooking Time: 30 minutes

Serving: 4

Ingredients:

2 lbs butternut squash, chopped

1 onion, chopped

3/4 cup water

1 tsp garlic powder

1 tsp chili powder

1 tbsp pumpkin pie spice

1 tsp dried oregano

Directions:

Add all ingredients into the Pressure Pot and stir well.

Seal pot with a lid and select manual high for 3 minutes.

Release pressure using the quick-release method than open the lid.

Stir and serve.

Nutrition:

Calories 123, Carbohydrates 31g, Protein 2.9g, Fat 0.6g, Sugar 6.5g, Sodium 19mg.

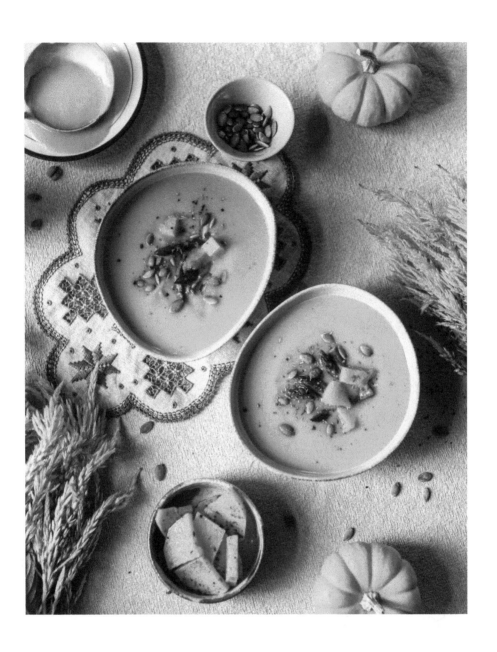

Green Pea Mash

Preparation Time: 5 minutes | Cooking Time: 30 minutes

Serving: 4

Ingredients:

1 cup green peas, frozen and thawed

1 cup vegetable stock

1 cup heavy cream

2 tbsp butter

Pepper

Salt

Directions:

Add butter into the Pressure Pot and set the pot on sauté mode.

Add peas and sauté for 2 minutes.

Add stock, heavy cream, and salt. Stir well.

Seal pot with lid and cook on high for 6 minutes.

Allow releasing pressure naturally for 10 minutes then release using the quick release method.

Puree the pea's mixture using an immersion blender until smooth.

Serve and enjoy.

Nutrition:

Calories 248, Carbohydrates 8.8g, Protein 3.5g, Fat 23g, Sugar 3.5g, Sodium 363mg.

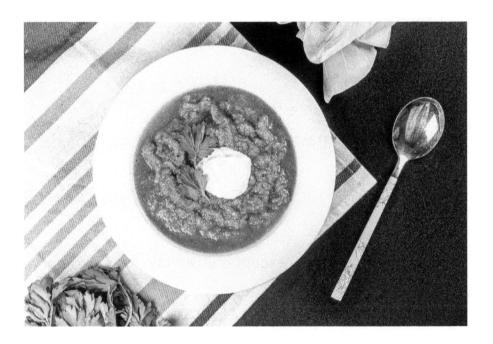

Black Eyed Peas

Preparation Time: 5 minutes | Cooking Time: 30 minutes

Serving: 4

Ingredients:

1/2 cup dry black-eyed peas

1 tbsp butter

1/2 cup onion, chopped

1 cup Swiss chard

1 1/4 cup vegetable stock

1/2 cup can tomato

1/2 tsp pepper

1/2 tsp salt

Directions:

Add all ingredients except butter into the pot and stir well.

Add butter on top. Seal pot with lid and cook on high for 15 minutes.

Allow releasing pressure naturally for 10 minutes then release using the quick release method.

Stir well and serve.

Nutrition:

Calories 117, Carbohydrates 20.6g, Protein 6.9g, Fat 4.7g, Sugar 3.8g, Sodium 835mg.

Pressure Pot Taco Meat

Preparation Time: 5 minutes | Cooking Time: 20 minutes

Serving: 4

Ingredients:

2 pounds ground beef

2 onions, diced

3 bell peppers (any color, diced)

2 packets of taco seasoning

1 cup of water

Directions:

Press the Sauté button on the Pressure Pot and stir in the beef and ground onions.

Allow to brown for 3 minutes while stirring constantly.

Add the rest of the ingredients.

Close Pressure Pot, press the Manual cook button, choose high settings, and set time to 10 minutes.

Once done cooking, do a QPR.

Serve and enjoy.

Nutrition:

Calories 612, Carbohydrates 8.3g, Protein 58.6g, Fat 36.8g, Sugar 2.6g, Sodium 158mg.

Beef Cheesy Potatoes

Preparation Time: 5 minutes | Cooking Time: 20 minutes

Serving: 4

Ingredients:

1 ½ pounds ground beef

6 large potatoes, peeled and chopped

2 cups cheddar cheese, shredded

¾ cup chicken broth

1 tablespoon Italian seasoning mix

Salt and pepper to taste

Directions:

Press the Sauté button on the Pressure Pot and stir in the beef. Brown the meat until some of the oil has rendered.

Add the rest of the ingredients.

Close Pressure Pot, press the Manual button, choose high settings, and set the time to 20 minutes.

Once done cooking, do a QPR.

Serve and enjoy.

Nutrition:

Calories 806, Carbohydrates 66.8g, Protein 53.4g, Fat 35.6g, Sugar 3.5g, Sodium 609mg.

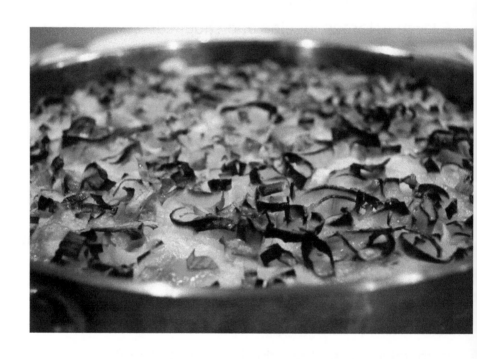

Sweet Potato Chili Recipe

Preparation Time: 5 minutes | Cooking Time: 30 minutes

Serving: 4

Ingredients:

1 teaspoon olive oil

1 onion, diced

3 cloves of garlic, minced

½ pound ground pork

1-pound ground beef

1 large sweet potato, peeled and cut into ½" pieces

3 celery stalks, sliced

3 ½ cups crushed tomatoes

1 tablespoon Worcestershire sauce

1 teaspoon cumin

1 teaspoon chili powder

Salt and pepper to taste

Directions:

Press the Sauté button on the Pressure Pot and heat the olive oil. Sauté the onion and garlic until fragrant.

Stir in the pork and beef and allow to brown for 5 minutes.

Add the rest of the ingredients.

Close Pressure Pot, press the Manual button, choose high settings, and set the time to 20 minutes.

Once done cooking, do a QPR.

Serve and enjoy.

Nutrition:

Calories 447, Carbohydrates 16.4g, Protein 36.9g, Fat 25.9g, Sugar 4.1g, Sodium 172mg.

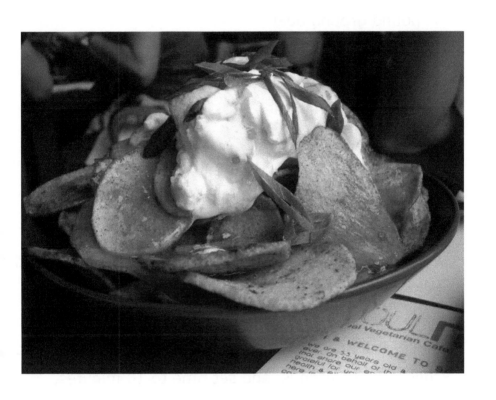

Pressure Pot Stuffed Peppers

Preparation Time: 5 minutes | Cooking Time: 40 minutes

Serving: 4

Ingredients:

½ pound ground beef

1/3 cup diced onions

1 ½ cup spaghetti sauce

½ teaspoon garlic salt

2 cups cooked rice

8 bell peppers, cut the top, and remove the seeds

1 cup mozzarella cheese, shredded

Directions:

Press the Sauté button on the Pressure Pot and add the beef and onions. Stir constantly.

Stir in the spaghetti sauce and season with garlic salt.

Close Pressure Pot, press the Manual cook button, choose high settings, and set time to 10 minutes.

Once done cooking, do a QPR.

Transfer into a bowl and add the cooked rice. Stir to combine. Pack the mixture into hollow bell peppers and top with mozzarella cheese.

Place a trivet in the Pressure Pot and pour water. Place the stuffed bell peppers on the trivet and close the lid. Press the Steam button and cook for 10 minutes.

Serve and enjoy.

Nutrition:

Calories 265, Carbohydrates 32g, Protein 12g, Fat 9g, Sugar 10g, Sodium 930mg.

Braised Brisket

Preparation Time: 5 minutes | Cooking Time: 30 minutes

Serving: 4

Ingredients:

2 pounds beef brisket, cut into 4 pieces

Salt and pepper to taste

2 cups sliced onion

½ cup of water

2 tablespoons tomato paste

2 tablespoons Worcestershire sauce

2 teaspoons liquid smoke

Directions:

Put all ingredients in the Pressure Pot. Mix all ingredients to combine everything.

Close Pressure Pot, press pressure cook button, choose high settings and set time to 60 minutes.

Once done cooking, do a QPR.

Serve and enjoy.

Nutrition:

Calories 490, Carbohydrates 9.9g, Protein 34.5g, Fat 33.9g, Sugar 4.8g, Sodium 885mg.

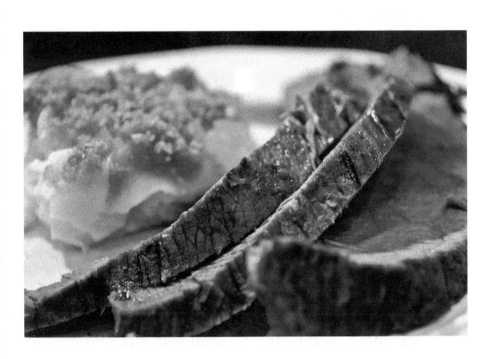

Pressure Pot Corned Beef and Cabbages

Preparation Time: 5 minutes | Cooking Time: 30 minutes

Serving: 4

Ingredients:

6 cloves of garlic, chopped

1 onion, quartered

2 ½ pounds corned beef brisket, cut in large slices

12-oz. beer

2 cups of water

3 carrots, roughly chopped

2 potatoes, chopped

1 head cabbage, cut into four pieces

Directions:

In the Pressure Pot, place the garlic, onion, corned beef brisket, beer, and water. Season with salt and pepper to taste.

Close Pressure Pot, press the Manual button, choose high settings, and set time to 50 minutes.

Once done cooking, do a QPR.

Open the lid and take out the meat. Shred the meat using a fork and place it back into the Pressure Pot.

Stir in the vegetables.

Close the lid and seal the vent and press the Manual button. Cook for another 10 minutes. Do QPR.

Serve and enjoy.

Nutrition:

Calories 758, Carbohydrates 45.8g, Protein 43.1g, Fat 44.7g, Sugar 8.7g, Sodium 940mg.

Beer Mustard Ham

Preparation Time: 5 minutes | Cooking Time: 60 minutes

Serving: 10-12

Ingredients:

½ teaspoon ground black pepper

3-pound bone-in ham chunk

2 bottles of beer

¾ cup Dijon mustard

4 sprigs of rosemary

Directions:

Take your Pressure Pot and place it over a dry kitchen platform.

Open the lid and add the ham. Pour the beer and add the mustard, pepper, and rosemary.

Lock the top lid and make sure that the valve is sealed properly.

Select "Meat/Stew" cooking function. Set the cooking time to 60 minutes.

Your Pressure Pot will start building the pressure and begin the cooking cycle after a sufficient level of pressure is reached.

After the cooking time is over, press the "Cancel" setting, and then press "NPR" for the natural release of the internal pressure. It takes around 10 minutes to release the pressure naturally.

Open the top lid, slice the meat, and add back to the pot, let it infuse the flavors for a few minutes.

Transfer the meat to your serving plates and drizzle the remaining sauce on top.

Serve and enjoy the recipe.

Nutrition:

Calories 143, Total Carbohydrates 12g, Fiber 0.5g, Saturated Fat 23g, Trans Fat 0g, Protein 6g, Sodium 231g.

Green Bean Mushroom Pork

Preparation Time: 5 minutes | Cooking Time: 30 minutes

Serving: 4

Ingredients:

½ cup onions, diced

3 tablespoons garlic, minced

8 ounces white button mushrooms, sliced

4 cups green beans, halved

1 tablespoon olive oil

4 pork chops

2 cups chicken broth

¼ cup honey

½ cup Dijon mustard

Pepper and salt as per your taste preference

1 tablespoon cornstarch + 2 tablespoons water

Directions:

Take your Pressure Pot and place it over a dry kitchen platform.

Open the lid and select the "Sauté" cooking function.

Add the oil and chops into the pot; cook to soften and sear evenly.

Add the onion and garlic; sauté for a few minutes.

Add the remaining ingredients except for the cornstarch mix; gently stir.

Lock the top lid and make sure that the valve is sealed properly.

Select "Meat/Stew" cooking function. Set the cooking time to 30 minutes.

Your Pressure Pot will start building the pressure and begin the cooking cycle after a sufficient level of pressure is reached.

After the cooking time is over, press the "Cancel" setting, and then press "NPR" for the natural release of the internal pressure. It takes around 10 minutes to release the pressure naturally.

Open the top lid, mix in the cornstarch mix, and stir thoroughly.

Transfer the meal to your serving bowls.

Serve and enjoy the recipe.

Nutrition:

Calories 364, Total Carbohydrates 10g, Fiber 3g, Saturated Fat 18g, Trans Fat 0g, Protein 27g, Sodium 534g.

Corned Beef

Preparation time: 10 minutes | Cooking Time: 60 minutes | Servings: 6

Ingredients:

4 pounds beef brisket

2 oranges, sliced

2 garlic cloves, peeled and minced

2 yellow onions, peeled and sliced thin

11 ounces celery, sliced thin

1 tablespoon dried dill

3 bay leaves

4 cinnamon sticks, cut into halves

Salt and ground black pepper, to taste

17 ounces of water

Directions:

Put the beef in a bowl, add some water to cover, set aside to soak for a few hours, drain and transfer to the Pressure Pot.

Add the celery, orange slices, onions, garlic, bay leaves, dill, cinnamon, dill, salt, pepper, and water. Stir, cover the Pressure Pot and cook on the Meat/Stew setting for 50 minutes.

Release the pressure, set the beef aside to cool for 5 minutes, transfer to a cutting board, slice, and divide among plates.

Drizzle the juice and vegetables from the Pressure Pot over beef and serve.

Nutrition:

Calories 251, Fat 3.14g, Fiber 0g, Carbs 1g, Protein 7g.

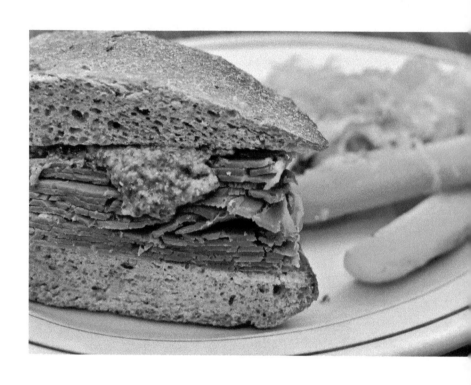

Beef Bourguignon

Preparation time: 15 minutes | Cooking Time: 30 minutes | Servings: 6

Ingredients:

10 pounds round steak, cut into small cubes

2 carrots, peeled and sliced

½ cup beef stock

1 cup dry red wine

3 bacon slices, chopped

8 ounces mushrooms, cut into quarters

2 tablespoons white flour

12 pearl onions

2 garlic cloves, peeled and minced

¼ teaspoon dried basil

Salt and ground black pepper, to taste

Directions:

Set the Pressure Pot on Sauté mode, add the bacon, and brown it for 2 minutes.

Add the beef pieces, stir, and brown for 5 minutes.

Add the flour and stir very well.

Add the salt, pepper, wine, stock, onions, garlic, and basil, stir, cover, and cook on the Meat/Stew setting for 20 minutes.

Release the pressure, uncover the Pressure Pot, add the mushrooms and carrots, cover the Pressure Pot again, and cook on the Manual setting for 5 minutes.

Release the pressure again, divide the beef bourguignon among plates, and serve.

Nutrition:

Calories 442, Fat 17.2g, Fiber 3g, Carbs 16g, Protein 39g.

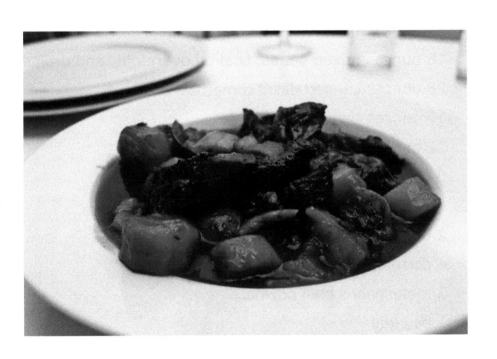

Beef Chili

Preparation time: 10 minutes | Cooking Time: 40 minutes | Servings: 6

Ingredients:

1½ pounds ground beef

1 sweet onion, peeled and chopped

Salt and ground black pepper, to taste

16 ounces mixed beans, soaked overnight, and drained

28 ounces canned diced tomatoes

17 ounces beef stock

12 ounces beer

6 garlic cloves, peeled and chopped

7 jalapeño peppers, diced

2 tablespoons vegetable oil

4 carrots, peeled and chopped

3 tablespoons chili powder

1 bay leaf

1 teaspoon chili powder

Directions:

Set the Pressure Pot on Sauté mode, add half of the oil, and heat it.

Add the beef, stir, brown for 8 minutes, and transfer to a bowl.

Add the rest of the oil to the Pressure Pot and heat it.

Add the carrots, onion, jalapeños, and garlic, stir, and sauté for 4 minutes.

Add the beer and tomatoes and stir.

Add the beans, bay leaf, stock, chili powder, chili powder, salt, pepper, and beef, stir, cover and cook on the Bean/Chili setting for 25 minutes.

Release the pressure naturally, uncover the Pressure Pot, stir chili, transfer to bowls, and serve.

Nutrition:

Calories 272, Fat 5g, Fiber 0g, Carbs 32g, Protein 25g.

Chili Con Carne

Preparation time: 10 minutes | Cooking Time: 30 minutes | Servings: 4

Ingredients:

1-pound ground beef

1 yellow onion, peeled and chopped

4 tablespoons extra virgin olive oil

Salt and ground black pepper, to taste

2 garlic cloves, peeled and minced

1 bay leaf

4 ounces kidney beans, soaked overnight and drained

1 teaspoon tomato paste

8 ounces canned diced tomatoes

1 tablespoon chili powder

½ teaspoon cumin

5 ounces of water

Directions:

Set the Pressure Pot on Sauté mode, add 1 tablespoon oil, and heat it.

Add the meat, brown for a few minutes, and transfer to a bowl.

Add the rest of the oil to the Pressure Pot and also heat it.

Add the onion and garlic, stir, and cook for 3 minutes.

Return the beef to the pot, add the bay leaf, beans, tomato paste, tomatoes, chili powder, cumin, salt, pepper, and water, stir, cover, and cook on the Bean/Chili setting for 18 minutes.

Release the pressure, uncover the Pressure Pot, discard bay leaf, divide chili among bowls, and serve.

Nutrition:

Calories 256, Fat 8g, Fiber 1g, Carbs 22g, Protein 25g.

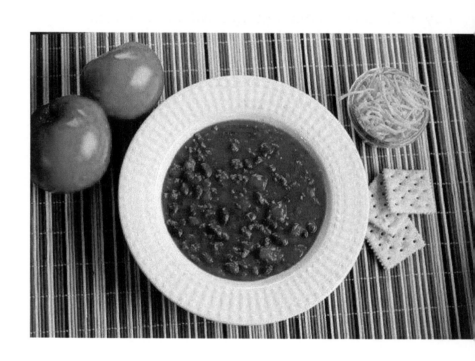

Beef Curry

Preparation time: 10 minutes | Cooking Time: 20 minutes | Servings: 4

Ingredients:

2 pounds beef steak, cubed

2 tablespoons extra virgin olive oil

3 potatoes, diced

1 tablespoon Dijon mustard

2½ tablespoons curry powder

2 yellow onions, peeled and chopped

2 garlic cloves, peeled and minced

10 ounces canned coconut milk

2 tablespoons tomato sauce

Salt and ground black pepper, to taste

Directions:

Set the Pressure Pot on Sauté mode, add the oil, and heat it.

Add the onions and garlic, stir and cook for 4 minutes.

Add the potatoes and mustard, stir, and cook for 1 minute.

Add the beef, stir, and brown on all sides.

Add the curry powder, salt, and pepper, stir, and cook for 2 minutes.

Add the coconut milk and tomato sauce, stir, cover the Pressure Pot, and cook on the Meat/Stew setting for 10 minutes.

Release the pressure, uncover the Pressure Pot, divide curry among plates, and serve.

Nutrition:

Calories 434, Fat 20g, Fiber 2.9g, Carbs 14g, Protein: 27.5g.

Beef Stroganoff

Preparation time: 10 minutes | Cooking Time: 25 minutes | Servings: 4

Ingredients:

10 pounds beef, cut into small cubes

1 yellow onion, peeled and chopped

2½ tablespoons vegetable oil

1½ tablespoons white flour

2 garlic cloves, peeled and minced

4 ounces mushrooms, sliced

1½ tablespoon tomato paste

Salt and ground black pepper, to taste

3 tablespoons Worcestershire sauce

13 ounces beef stock

8 ounces sour cream

Egg noodles, already cooked, for serving

Directions:

Put the beef, salt, pepper, and flour in a bowl and toss to coat.

Set the Pressure Pot on Sauté mode, add the oil, and heat it.

Add the meat and brown it on all sides.

Add the onion, garlic, mushrooms, Worcestershire sauce, stock, and tomato paste, stir well, cover the Pressure Pot and cook on the Meat/Stew setting for 20 minutes.

Release the pressure, uncover the Pressure Pot, add the sour cream, more salt, and pepper, stir well, divide among plates on top of egg noodles and serve.

Nutrition:

Calories 335, Fat 18.4g, Fiber 1.3g, Carbs 22.5g, Protein 20.1g.

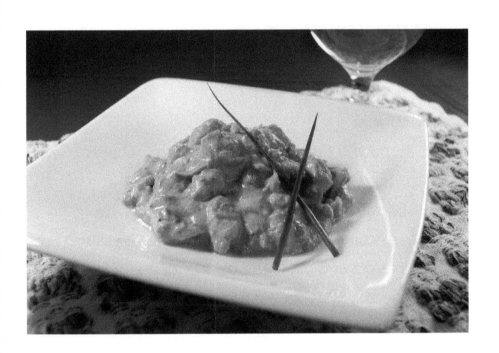

Moist Cream Cheese Muffins

Preparation Time: 10 minutes | Cooking Time: 20 minutes | Servings: 5

Ingredients:

1 egg

1/4 cup Erythritol

4 oz cream cheese

1/2 tsp ground cinnamon

1/4 tsp vanilla

Directions:

In a bowl, beat together cream cheese, vanilla, Erythritol, and eggs until fluffy.

Pour batter into the silicone muffin molds.

Place silicone muffin molds into the Pressure Pot air fryer basket and place the basket in the pot.

Seal the pot with an air fryer lid and select bake mode and cook at 350° F for 20 minutes.

Serve and enjoy.

Nutrition:

Calories 93, Fat 8g, Carbohydrates 11g, Sugar 12g, Protein 2g, Cholesterol 55mg.

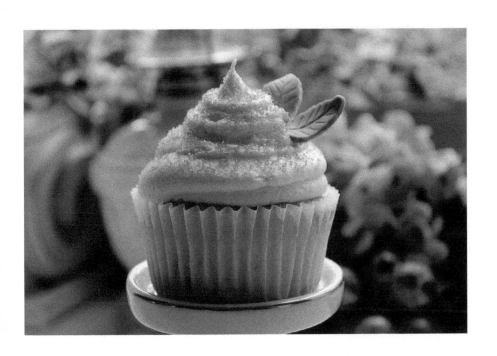

Parmesan Salmon

Preparation Time: 10 minutes | Cooking Time: 15 minutes | Servings: 4

Ingredients:

4 salmon fillets

1/4 cup parmesan cheese, grated

1/4 cup walnuts

1 tsp olive oil

1 tbsp lemon rind

Pepper

Salt

Directions:

Line Pressure Pot air fryer basket with parchment paper or foil.

Place salmon in the air fryer basket and place basket in the pot.

Add walnuts into the food processor and process until finely ground.

Mix ground walnuts with cheese, oil, and lemon rind. Stir well.

Spread walnut mixture over the salmon fillets and press gently.

Seal the pot with an air fryer lid and select bake mode and cook at 400° F for 15 minutes.

Serve and enjoy.

Nutrition:

Calories 420, Fat 26g, Carbohydrates 2g, Sugar 0.3g, Protein 45g, Cholesterol 97mg.

Bok Choy And Butter Sauce

Preparation time: 20 minutes | Cooking Time: 15 minutes | Servings: 4

Ingredients:

2 bok choy heads; trimmed and cut into strips

1 tbsp. Butter; melted

2 tbsp. Chicken stock

1 tsp. Lemon juice

1 tbsp. Olive oil

A pinch of salt and black pepper

Directions:

In a pan that fits your air fryer, mix all the ingredients, toss, introduce the pan in the air fryer, and cook at 380°F for 15 minutes.

Divide between plates and serve as a side dish

Nutrition:

Calories 141, Fat 3, Fiber 2g, Carbs 4g, Protein 3g.

Lightning Source UK Ltd.
Milton Keynes UK
UKHW020806180621
385732UK00001B/106